PHYSIO JOURNAL

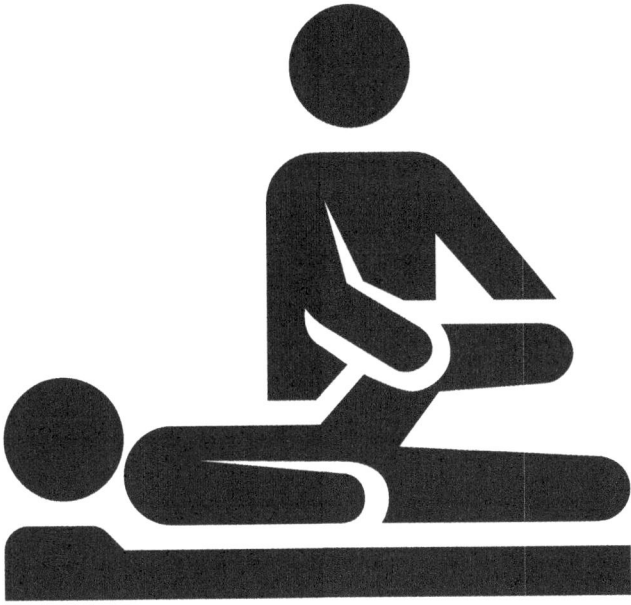

THIS NOTEBOOK BELONGS TO

....

....

....

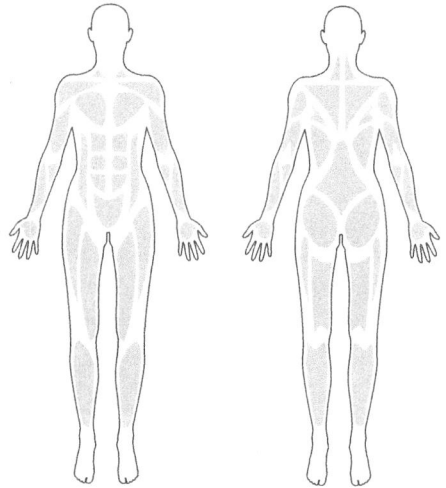 DATE	CLIENT CONDITIONS					
TIME	HEALTH	1	2	3	4	5
CLIENT	ENERGY	1	2	3	4	5
AGE	ACTIVITY	1	2	3	4	5
GENDER	SLEEP	1	2	3	4	5

ANALYSIS OF SYMPTOM

DESCRIPTION	PAIN AREA
	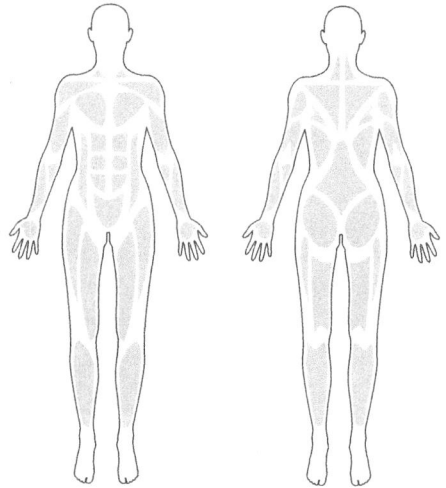

PAIN LEVEL

1	2	3	4	5	6	7	8	9	10

EXERCISE PLAN

	DESCRIPTION	DURATION / FREQUENCY
1		
2		
3		
4		
5		
6		
7		
8		
9		

📅 DATE		CLIENT CONDITIONS					
🕐 TIME		〰️ HEALTH	1	2	3	4	5
👤 CLIENT		⚡ ENERGY	1	2	3	4	5
📅 AGE		🏃 ACTIVITY	1	2	3	4	5
⚧ GENDER		🌙 SLEEP	1	2	3	4	5

ANALYSIS OF SYMPTOM

DESCRIPTION	PAIN AREA

PAIN LEVEL

1	2	3	4	5	6	7	8	9	10

EXERCISE PLAN

	DESCRIPTION	DURATION / FREQUENCY
1		
2		
3		
4		
5		
6		
7		
8		
9		

📅 DATE		CLIENT CONDITIONS					
🕐 TIME		💓 HEALTH	1	2	3	4	5
👤 CLIENT		⚡ ENERGY	1	2	3	4	5
📅 AGE		🏃 ACTIVITY	1	2	3	4	5
⚥ GENDER		🌙 SLEEP	1	2	3	4	5

ANALYSIS OF SYMPTOM

DESCRIPTION	PAIN AREA

PAIN LEVEL

1	2	3	4	5	6	7	8	9	10

EXERCISE PLAN

	DESCRIPTION	DURATION / FREQUENCY
1		
2		
3		
4		
5		
6		
7		
8		
9		

DATE	CLIENT CONDITIONS					
TIME	HEALTH	1	2	3	4	5
CLIENT	ENERGY	1	2	3	4	5
AGE	ACTIVITY	1	2	3	4	5
GENDER	SLEEP	1	2	3	4	5

ANALYSIS OF SYMPTOM

DESCRIPTION	PAIN AREA

PAIN LEVEL

1	2	3	4	5	6	7	8	9	10

EXERCISE PLAN

	DESCRIPTION	DURATION / FREQUENCY
1		
2		
3		
4		
5		
6		
7		
8		
9		

📅 DATE		**CLIENT CONDITIONS**					
🕐 TIME		💓 HEALTH	1	2	3	4	5
🧍 CLIENT		⚡ ENERGY	1	2	3	4	5
📅 AGE		🏃 ACTIVITY	1	2	3	4	5
⚥ GENDER		🌙 SLEEP	1	2	3	4	5

ANALYSIS OF SYMPTOM

DESCRIPTION	PAIN AREA
	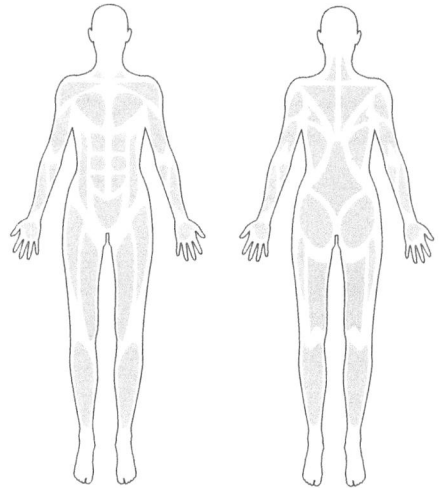

PAIN LEVEL

1	2	3	4	5	6	7	8	9	10

EXERCISE PLAN

	DESCRIPTION	DURATION / FREQUENCY
1		
2		
3		
4		
5		
6		
7		
8		
9		

DATE	CLIENT CONDITIONS					
TIME	HEALTH	1	2	3	4	5
CLIENT	ENERGY	1	2	3	4	5
AGE	ACTIVITY	1	2	3	4	5
GENDER	SLEEP	1	2	3	4	5

ANALYSIS OF SYMPTOM

DESCRIPTION	PAIN AREA

PAIN LEVEL

1	2	3	4	5	6	7	8	9	10

EXERCISE PLAN

	DESCRIPTION	DURATION / FREQUENCY
1		
2		
3		
4		
5		
6		
7		
8		
9		

📅 DATE		CLIENT CONDITIONS					
🕐 TIME		❤️ HEALTH	1	2	3	4	5
👤 CLIENT		⚡ ENERGY	1	2	3	4	5
📅 AGE		🏃 ACTIVITY	1	2	3	4	5
⚤ GENDER		🌙 SLEEP	1	2	3	4	5

ANALYSIS OF SYMPTOM

DESCRIPTION	PAIN AREA

PAIN LEVEL

1	2	3	4	5	6	7	8	9	10

EXERCISE PLAN

	DESCRIPTION	DURATION / FREQUENCY
1		
2		
3		
4		
5		
6		
7		
8		
9		

📅 DATE		CLIENT CONDITIONS					
🕐 TIME							
👤 CLIENT	❤️ HEALTH	1	2	3	4	5	
	⚡ ENERGY	1	2	3	4	5	
📅 AGE	🏃 ACTIVITY	1	2	3	4	5	
⚥ GENDER	🌙 SLEEP	1	2	3	4	5	

ANALYSIS OF SYMPTOM

DESCRIPTION	PAIN AREA

PAIN LEVEL

1	2	3	4	5	6	7	8	9	10

EXERCISE PLAN

	DESCRIPTION	DURATION / FREQUENCY
1		
2		
3		
4		
5		
6		
7		
8		
9		

📅 **DATE**		**CLIENT CONDITIONS**					

📅 **DATE**
🕐 **TIME**
👤 **CLIENT**
📅 **AGE**
⚤ **GENDER**

CLIENT CONDITIONS

💓 HEALTH	1	2	3	4	5
⚡ ENERGY	1	2	3	4	5
🏃 ACTIVITY	1	2	3	4	5
🌙 SLEEP	1	2	3	4	5

ANALYSIS OF SYMPTOM

DESCRIPTION	PAIN AREA
	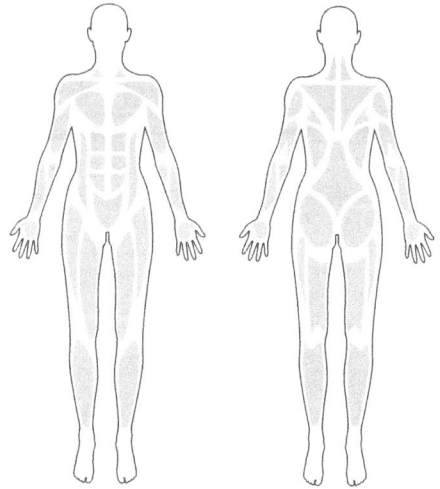

PAIN LEVEL

1	2	3	4	5	6	7	8	9	10

EXERCISE PLAN

	DESCRIPTION	DURATION / FREQUENCY
1		
2		
3		
4		
5		
6		
7		
8		
9		

DATE		CLIENT CONDITIONS					
TIME		HEALTH	1	2	3	4	5
CLIENT		ENERGY	1	2	3	4	5
AGE		ACTIVITY	1	2	3	4	5
GENDER		SLEEP	1	2	3	4	5

ANALYSIS OF SYMPTOM

DESCRIPTION	PAIN AREA

PAIN LEVEL

1	2	3	4	5	6	7	8	9	10

EXERCISE PLAN

	DESCRIPTION	DURATION / FREQUENCY
1		
2		
3		
4		
5		
6		
7		
8		
9		

📅 DATE	
🕐 TIME	
👤 CLIENT	
📆 AGE	
⚥ GENDER	

CLIENT CONDITIONS

💗 HEALTH	1	2	3	4	5
⚡ ENERGY	1	2	3	4	5
🏃 ACTIVITY	1	2	3	4	5
🌙 SLEEP	1	2	3	4	5

ANALYSIS OF SYMPTOM

DESCRIPTION	PAIN AREA

PAIN LEVEL

1	2	3	4	5	6	7	8	9	10

EXERCISE PLAN

	DESCRIPTION	DURATION / FREQUENCY
1		
2		
3		
4		
5		
6		
7		
8		
9		

📅 DATE	
🕐 TIME	
👤 CLIENT	
📅 AGE	
⚥ GENDER	

CLIENT CONDITIONS

♥ HEALTH	1 2 3 4 5
⚡ ENERGY	1 2 3 4 5
🏃 ACTIVITY	1 2 3 4 5
🌙 SLEEP	1 2 3 4 5

ANALYSIS OF SYMPTOM

DESCRIPTION	PAIN AREA

PAIN LEVEL

1 2 3 4 5 6 7 8 9 10

EXERCISE PLAN

	DESCRIPTION	DURATION / FREQUENCY
1		
2		
3		
4		
5		
6		
7		
8		
9		

📅 DATE	
🕐 TIME	
👤 CLIENT	
📅 AGE	
⚥ GENDER	

CLIENT CONDITIONS

❤️ HEALTH	1	2	3	4	5
⚡ ENERGY	1	2	3	4	5
🏃 ACTIVITY	1	2	3	4	5
🌙 SLEEP	1	2	3	4	5

ANALYSIS OF SYMPTOM

DESCRIPTION	PAIN AREA
	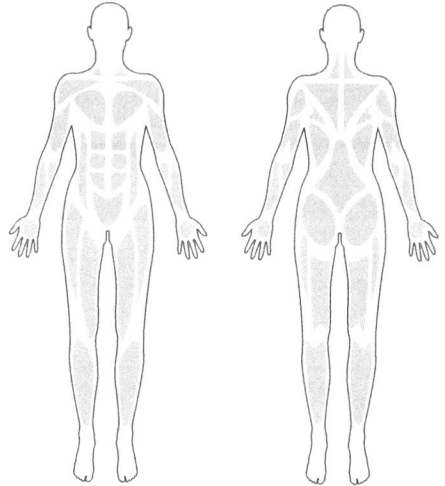

PAIN LEVEL

1	2	3	4	5	6	7	8	9	10

EXERCISE PLAN

	DESCRIPTION	DURATION / FREQUENCY
1		
2		
3		
4		
5		
6		
7		
8		
9		

DATE

TIME

CLIENT

AGE

GENDER

CLIENT CONDITIONS					
HEALTH	1	2	3	4	5
ENERGY	1	2	3	4	5
ACTIVITY	1	2	3	4	5
SLEEP	1	2	3	4	5

ANALYSIS OF SYMPTOM

DESCRIPTION	PAIN AREA

PAIN LEVEL

1	2	3	4	5	6	7	8	9	10

EXERCISE PLAN

	DESCRIPTION	DURATION / FREQUENCY
1		
2		
3		
4		
5		
6		
7		
8		
9		

📅 DATE		CLIENT CONDITIONS	
🕐 TIME		❤️ HEALTH	(1 | 2 | 3 | 4 | 5)
👤 CLIENT		⚡ ENERGY	(1 | 2 | 3 | 4 | 5)
📅 AGE		🏃 ACTIVITY	(1 | 2 | 3 | 4 | 5)
⚧ GENDER		🌙 SLEEP	(1 | 2 | 3 | 4 | 5)

ANALYSIS OF SYMPTOM

DESCRIPTION	PAIN AREA

PAIN LEVEL

(1 | 2 | 3 | 4 | 5 | 6 | 7 | 8 | 9 | 10)

EXERCISE PLAN

	DESCRIPTION	DURATION / FREQUENCY
1		
2		
3		
4		
5		
6		
7		
8		
9		

	DATE		CLIENT CONDITIONS	

DATE	
TIME	
CLIENT	
AGE	
GENDER	

CLIENT CONDITIONS

HEALTH		1	2	3	4	5	
ENERGY		1	2	3	4	5	
ACTIVITY		1	2	3	4	5	
SLEEP		1	2	3	4	5	

ANALYSIS OF SYMPTOM

DESCRIPTION	PAIN AREA

PAIN LEVEL

1	2	3	4	5	6	7	8	9	10

EXERCISE PLAN

	DESCRIPTION	DURATION / FREQUENCY
1		
2		
3		
4		
5		
6		
7		
8		
9		

📅 DATE		CLIENT CONDITIONS	
🕐 TIME		💓 HEALTH	1 2 3 4 5
👤 CLIENT		⚡ ENERGY	1 2 3 4 5
📅 AGE		🏃 ACTIVITY	1 2 3 4 5
⚧ GENDER		🌙 SLEEP	1 2 3 4 5

ANALYSIS OF SYMPTOM

DESCRIPTION	PAIN AREA
	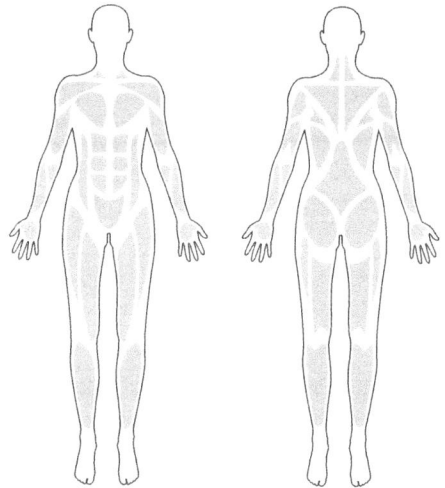

PAIN LEVEL

1	2	3	4	5	6	7	8	9	10

EXERCISE PLAN

	DESCRIPTION	DURATION / FREQUENCY
1		
2		
3		
4		
5		
6		
7		
8		
9		

📅 DATE		CLIENT CONDITIONS					
🕐 TIME		❤️‍🩹 HEALTH	1	2	3	4	5
👤 CLIENT		⚡ ENERGY	1	2	3	4	5
📅 AGE		🏃 ACTIVITY	1	2	3	4	5
⚥ GENDER		🌙 SLEEP	1	2	3	4	5

ANALYSIS OF SYMPTOM

DESCRIPTION	PAIN AREA

PAIN LEVEL

1	2	3	4	5	6	7	8	9	10

EXERCISE PLAN

	DESCRIPTION	DURATION / FREQUENCY
1		
2		
3		
4		
5		
6		
7		
8		
9		

📅 DATE		**CLIENT CONDITIONS**					
🕐 TIME		💗 HEALTH	1	2	3	4	5
👤 CLIENT		⚡ ENERGY	1	2	3	4	5
📅 AGE		🏃 ACTIVITY	1	2	3	4	5
⚧ GENDER		🌙 SLEEP	1	2	3	4	5

ANALYSIS OF SYMPTOM

DESCRIPTION	PAIN AREA

PAIN LEVEL

1	2	3	4	5	6	7	8	9	10

EXERCISE PLAN

	DESCRIPTION	DURATION / FREQUENCY
1		
2		
3		
4		
5		
6		
7		
8		
9		

📅 DATE		CLIENT CONDITIONS

📅 DATE	
🕐 TIME	
👤 CLIENT	
📅 AGE	
⚥ GENDER	

CLIENT CONDITIONS					
💓 HEALTH	1	2	3	4	5
⚡ ENERGY	1	2	3	4	5
🏃 ACTIVITY	1	2	3	4	5
🌙 SLEEP	1	2	3	4	5

ANALYSIS OF SYMPTOM

DESCRIPTION	PAIN AREA

PAIN LEVEL

1	2	3	4	5	6	7	8	9	10

EXERCISE PLAN

	DESCRIPTION	DURATION / FREQUENCY
1		
2		
3		
4		
5		
6		
7		
8		
9		

📅 DATE		CLIENT CONDITIONS					
🕐 TIME		💗 HEALTH	1	2	3	4	5
👤 CLIENT		⚡ ENERGY	1	2	3	4	5
📅 AGE		🏃 ACTIVITY	1	2	3	4	5
⚥ GENDER		🌙 SLEEP	1	2	3	4	5

ANALYSIS OF SYMPTOM

DESCRIPTION	PAIN AREA
	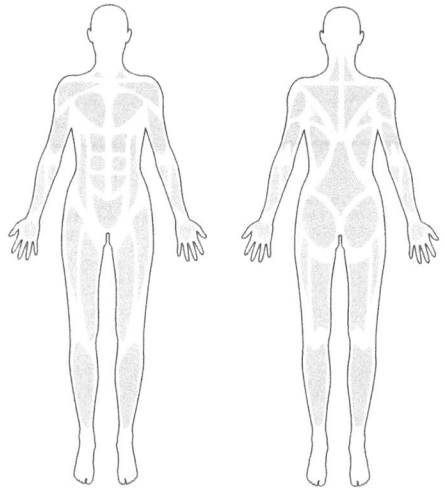

PAIN LEVEL

1	2	3	4	5	6	7	8	9	10

EXERCISE PLAN

	DESCRIPTION	DURATION / FREQUENCY
1		
2		
3		
4		
5		
6		
7		
8		
9		

📅 DATE		**CLIENT CONDITIONS**					
🕐 TIME		〜 HEALTH	1	2	3	4	5
👤 CLIENT		⚡ ENERGY	1	2	3	4	5
📅 AGE		🏃 ACTIVITY	1	2	3	4	5
⚤ GENDER		🌙 SLEEP	1	2	3	4	5

ANALYSIS OF SYMPTOM

DESCRIPTION	PAIN AREA

PAIN LEVEL

1	2	3	4	5	6	7	8	9	10

EXERCISE PLAN

	DESCRIPTION	DURATION / FREQUENCY
1		
2		
3		
4		
5		
6		
7		
8		
9		

📅 DATE		CLIENT CONDITIONS	
🕐 TIME		❤️ HEALTH	1 2 3 4 5
🧍 CLIENT		⚡ ENERGY	1 2 3 4 5
📅 AGE		🏃 ACTIVITY	1 2 3 4 5
⚧ GENDER		🌙 SLEEP	1 2 3 4 5

ANALYSIS OF SYMPTOM

DESCRIPTION	PAIN AREA

PAIN LEVEL

1	2	3	4	5	6	7	8	9	10

EXERCISE PLAN

	DESCRIPTION	DURATION / FREQUENCY
1		
2		
3		
4		
5		
6		
7		
8		
9		

📅 DATE		CLIENT CONDITIONS					
🕐 TIME		〰 HEALTH	1	2	3	4	5
👤 CLIENT		⚡ ENERGY	1	2	3	4	5
📅 AGE		🏃 ACTIVITY	1	2	3	4	5
⚥ GENDER		🌙 SLEEP	1	2	3	4	5

ANALYSIS OF SYMPTOM

DESCRIPTION	PAIN AREA

PAIN LEVEL

1	2	3	4	5	6	7	8	9	10

EXERCISE PLAN

	DESCRIPTION	DURATION / FREQUENCY
1		
2		
3		
4		
5		
6		
7		
8		
9		

📅 DATE		CLIENT CONDITIONS					
🕐 TIME		💓 HEALTH	1	2	3	4	5
👤 CLIENT		⚡ ENERGY	1	2	3	4	5
📅 AGE		🏃 ACTIVITY	1	2	3	4	5
⚥ GENDER		🌙 SLEEP	1	2	3	4	5

ANALYSIS OF SYMPTOM

DESCRIPTION	PAIN AREA
	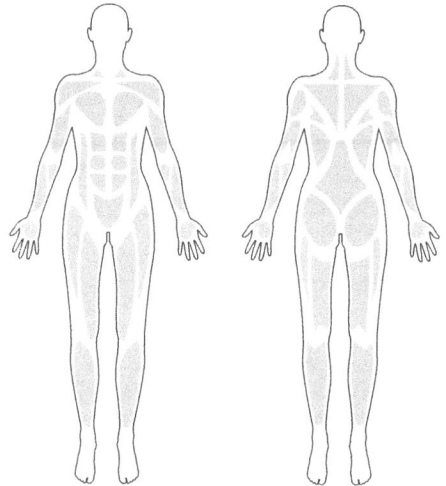

PAIN LEVEL

1	2	3	4	5	6	7	8	9	10

EXERCISE PLAN

	DESCRIPTION	DURATION / FREQUENCY
1		
2		
3		
4		
5		
6		
7		
8		
9		

	DATE		CLIENT CONDITIONS						
	TIME		HEALTH	1	2	3	4	5	
	CLIENT		ENERGY	1	2	3	4	5	
	AGE		ACTIVITY	1	2	3	4	5	
	GENDER		SLEEP	1	2	3	4	5	

ANALYSIS OF SYMPTOM

DESCRIPTION	PAIN AREA

PAIN LEVEL

1	2	3	4	5	6	7	8	9	10

EXERCISE PLAN

	DESCRIPTION	DURATION / FREQUENCY
1		
2		
3		
4		
5		
6		
7		
8		
9		

📅 DATE		CLIENT CONDITIONS	

📅 DATE	
🕐 TIME	
👤 CLIENT	
📅 AGE	
⚥ GENDER	

CLIENT CONDITIONS

💓 HEALTH	1 2 3 4 5
⚡ ENERGY	1 2 3 4 5
🏃 ACTIVITY	1 2 3 4 5
🌙 SLEEP	1 2 3 4 5

ANALYSIS OF SYMPTOM

DESCRIPTION	PAIN AREA

PAIN LEVEL

1 2 3 4 5 6 7 8 9 10

EXERCISE PLAN

	DESCRIPTION	DURATION / FREQUENCY
1		
2		
3		
4		
5		
6		
7		
8		
9		

	DATE		CLIENT CONDITIONS					

DATE		CLIENT CONDITIONS
TIME	HEALTH	1 2 3 4 5
CLIENT	ENERGY	1 2 3 4 5
AGE	ACTIVITY	1 2 3 4 5
GENDER	SLEEP	1 2 3 4 5

ANALYSIS OF SYMPTOM

DESCRIPTION	PAIN AREA

PAIN LEVEL

1 2 3 4 5 6 7 8 9 10

EXERCISE PLAN

	DESCRIPTION	DURATION / FREQUENCY
1		
2		
3		
4		
5		
6		
7		
8		
9		

DATE		**CLIENT CONDITIONS**					

DATE		**CLIENT CONDITIONS**
TIME		**HEALTH** — 1 2 3 4 5
CLIENT		**ENERGY** — 1 2 3 4 5
AGE		**ACTIVITY** — 1 2 3 4 5
GENDER		**SLEEP** — 1 2 3 4 5

ANALYSIS OF SYMPTOM

DESCRIPTION	PAIN AREA

PAIN LEVEL

1 2 3 4 5 6 7 8 9 10

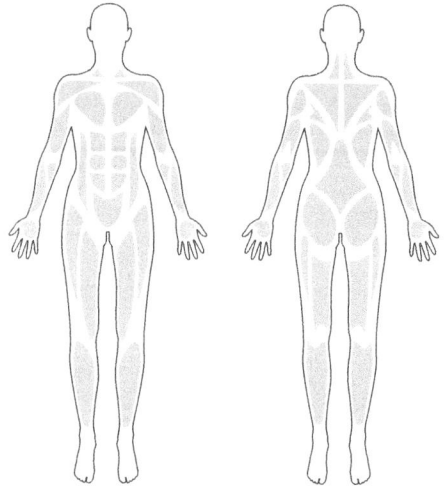

EXERCISE PLAN

	DESCRIPTION	DURATION / FREQUENCY
1		
2		
3		
4		
5		
6		
7		
8		
9		

📅 DATE		CLIENT CONDITIONS

📅 DATE	CLIENT CONDITIONS					
🕐 TIME	〰️ HEALTH	1	2	3	4	5
👤 CLIENT	⚡ ENERGY	1	2	3	4	5
📅 AGE	🏃 ACTIVITY	1	2	3	4	5
⚥ GENDER	🌙 SLEEP	1	2	3	4	5

ANALYSIS OF SYMPTOM

DESCRIPTION	PAIN AREA

PAIN LEVEL

1	2	3	4	5	6	7	8	9	10

EXERCISE PLAN

	DESCRIPTION	DURATION / FREQUENCY
1		
2		
3		
4		
5		
6		
7		
8		
9		

📅 DATE		CLIENT CONDITIONS	

📅 DATE
🕐 TIME
🧍 CLIENT
📅 AGE
⚥ GENDER

CLIENT CONDITIONS	
💓 HEALTH	1 2 3 4 5
⚡ ENERGY	1 2 3 4 5
🏃 ACTIVITY	1 2 3 4 5
🌙 SLEEP	1 2 3 4 5

ANALYSIS OF SYMPTOM

DESCRIPTION	PAIN AREA

PAIN LEVEL

1	2	3	4	5	6	7	8	9	10

EXERCISE PLAN

	DESCRIPTION	DURATION / FREQUENCY
1		
2		
3		
4		
5		
6		
7		
8		
9		

DATE		**CLIENT CONDITIONS**					

DATE
TIME
CLIENT
AGE
GENDER

CLIENT CONDITIONS

HEALTH	1	2	3	4	5
ENERGY	1	2	3	4	5
ACTIVITY	1	2	3	4	5
SLEEP	1	2	3	4	5

ANALYSIS OF SYMPTOM

DESCRIPTION	PAIN AREA

PAIN LEVEL

1	2	3	4	5	6	7	8	9	10

EXERCISE PLAN

	DESCRIPTION	DURATION / FREQUENCY
1		
2		
3		
4		
5		
6		
7		
8		
9		

	DATE		CLIENT CONDITIONS					

DATE	
TIME	
CLIENT	
AGE	
GENDER	

CLIENT CONDITIONS

HEALTH	1	2	3	4	5
ENERGY	1	2	3	4	5
ACTIVITY	1	2	3	4	5
SLEEP	1	2	3	4	5

ANALYSIS OF SYMPTOM

DESCRIPTION	PAIN AREA

PAIN LEVEL

1	2	3	4	5	6	7	8	9	10

EXERCISE PLAN

	DESCRIPTION	DURATION / FREQUENCY
1		
2		
3		
4		
5		
6		
7		
8		
9		

DATE		CLIENT CONDITIONS					
TIME		HEALTH	1	2	3	4	5
CLIENT		ENERGY	1	2	3	4	5
AGE		ACTIVITY	1	2	3	4	5
GENDER		SLEEP	1	2	3	4	5

ANALYSIS OF SYMPTOM

DESCRIPTION	PAIN AREA

PAIN LEVEL

1	2	3	4	5	6	7	8	9	10

EXERCISE PLAN

	DESCRIPTION	DURATION / FREQUENCY
1		
2		
3		
4		
5		
6		
7		
8		
9		

📅 DATE		CLIENT CONDITIONS					
🕐 TIME		〰️ HEALTH	1	2	3	4	5
👤 CLIENT		⚡ ENERGY	1	2	3	4	5
📅 AGE		🏃 ACTIVITY	1	2	3	4	5
⚥ GENDER		🌙 SLEEP	1	2	3	4	5

ANALYSIS OF SYMPTOM

DESCRIPTION	PAIN AREA

PAIN LEVEL

1	2	3	4	5	6	7	8	9	10

EXERCISE PLAN

	DESCRIPTION	DURATION / FREQUENCY
1		
2		
3		
4		
5		
6		
7		
8		
9		

	DATE		CLIENT CONDITIONS					

DATE	
TIME	
CLIENT	
AGE	
GENDER	

CLIENT CONDITIONS					
HEALTH	1	2	3	4	5
ENERGY	1	2	3	4	5
ACTIVITY	1	2	3	4	5
SLEEP	1	2	3	4	5

ANALYSIS OF SYMPTOM

DESCRIPTION	PAIN AREA

PAIN LEVEL

1	2	3	4	5	6	7	8	9	10

EXERCISE PLAN

	DESCRIPTION	DURATION / FREQUENCY
1		
2		
3		
4		
5		
6		
7		
8		
9		

📅 DATE		CLIENT CONDITIONS					
🕐 TIME		❤️ HEALTH	1	2	3	4	5
👤 CLIENT		⚡ ENERGY	1	2	3	4	5
📅 AGE		🏃 ACTIVITY	1	2	3	4	5
⚥ GENDER		🌙 SLEEP	1	2	3	4	5

ANALYSIS OF SYMPTOM

DESCRIPTION	PAIN AREA
	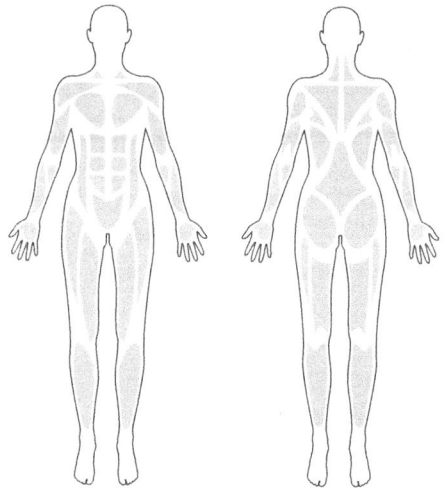

PAIN LEVEL

1	2	3	4	5	6	7	8	9	10

EXERCISE PLAN

	DESCRIPTION	DURATION / FREQUENCY
1		
2		
3		
4		
5		
6		
7		
8		
9		

DATE		CLIENT CONDITIONS					

DATE

TIME

CLIENT

AGE

GENDER

CLIENT CONDITIONS					
HEALTH	1	2	3	4	5
ENERGY	1	2	3	4	5
ACTIVITY	1	2	3	4	5
SLEEP	1	2	3	4	5

ANALYSIS OF SYMPTOM

DESCRIPTION	PAIN AREA

PAIN LEVEL

1	2	3	4	5	6	7	8	9	10

EXERCISE PLAN

	DESCRIPTION	DURATION / FREQUENCY
1		
2		
3		
4		
5		
6		
7		
8		
9		

📅 DATE		**CLIENT CONDITIONS**					

📅 **DATE**	
🕐 **TIME**	
👤 **CLIENT**	
📅 **AGE**	
⚥ **GENDER**	

CLIENT CONDITIONS					
〽️ HEALTH	1	2	3	4	5
⚡ ENERGY	1	2	3	4	5
🏃 ACTIVITY	1	2	3	4	5
🌙 SLEEP	1	2	3	4	5

ANALYSIS OF SYMPTOM

DESCRIPTION	PAIN AREA

PAIN LEVEL

1	2	3	4	5	6	7	8	9	10

EXERCISE PLAN

	DESCRIPTION	DURATION / FREQUENCY
1		
2		
3		
4		
5		
6		
7		
8		
9		

📅 DATE		**CLIENT CONDITIONS**					
🕐 TIME		💗 HEALTH	1	2	3	4	5
👤 CLIENT		⚡ ENERGY	1	2	3	4	5
📅 AGE		🏃 ACTIVITY	1	2	3	4	5
⚧ GENDER		🌙 SLEEP	1	2	3	4	5

ANALYSIS OF SYMPTOM

DESCRIPTION	PAIN AREA

PAIN LEVEL

1	2	3	4	5	6	7	8	9	10

EXERCISE PLAN

	DESCRIPTION	DURATION / FREQUENCY
1		
2		
3		
4		
5		
6		
7		
8		
9		

	DATE	
	TIME	
	CLIENT	
	AGE	
	GENDER	

CLIENT CONDITIONS

HEALTH	1	2	3	4	5	
ENERGY	1	2	3	4	5	
ACTIVITY	1	2	3	4	5	
SLEEP	1	2	3	4	5	

ANALYSIS OF SYMPTOM

DESCRIPTION	PAIN AREA
	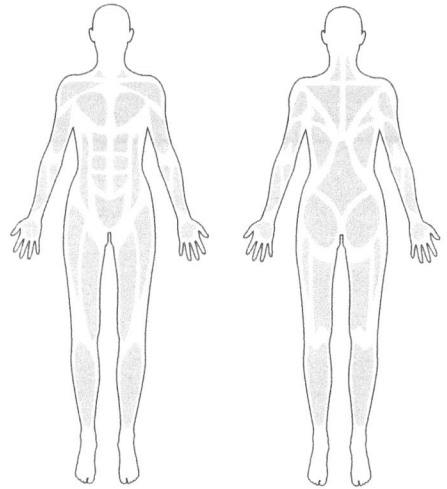

PAIN LEVEL

1	2	3	4	5	6	7	8	9	10

EXERCISE PLAN

	DESCRIPTION	DURATION / FREQUENCY
1		
2		
3		
4		
5		
6		
7		
8		
9		

📅 DATE	

| 🕐 TIME | |

| 👤 CLIENT | |

| 📅 AGE | |

| ⚥ GENDER | |

CLIENT CONDITIONS

❤️ HEALTH	1	2	3	4	5
⚡ ENERGY	1	2	3	4	5
🏃 ACTIVITY	1	2	3	4	5
🌙 SLEEP	1	2	3	4	5

ANALYSIS OF SYMPTOM

DESCRIPTION	PAIN AREA

PAIN LEVEL

1	2	3	4	5	6	7	8	9	10

EXERCISE PLAN

	DESCRIPTION	DURATION / FREQUENCY
1		
2		
3		
4		
5		
6		
7		
8		
9		

📅 DATE	
🕐 TIME	
👤 CLIENT	
📅 AGE	
⚥ GENDER	

CLIENT CONDITIONS

❤️ HEALTH	1	2	3	4	5
⚡ ENERGY	1	2	3	4	5
🏃 ACTIVITY	1	2	3	4	5
🌙 SLEEP	1	2	3	4	5

ANALYSIS OF SYMPTOM

DESCRIPTION	PAIN AREA

PAIN LEVEL

1	2	3	4	5	6	7	8	9	10

EXERCISE PLAN

	DESCRIPTION	DURATION / FREQUENCY
1		
2		
3		
4		
5		
6		
7		
8		
9		

	DATE		CLIENT CONDITIONS					
	TIME	HEALTH	1	2	3	4	5	
	CLIENT	ENERGY	1	2	3	4	5	
	AGE	ACTIVITY	1	2	3	4	5	
	GENDER	SLEEP	1	2	3	4	5	

ANALYSIS OF SYMPTOM

DESCRIPTION	PAIN AREA

PAIN LEVEL

1	2	3	4	5	6	7	8	9	10

EXERCISE PLAN

	DESCRIPTION	DURATION / FREQUENCY
1		
2		
3		
4		
5		
6		
7		
8		
9		

	DATE		CLIENT CONDITIONS	

DATE

TIME

CLIENT

AGE

GENDER

CLIENT CONDITIONS

HEALTH	1	2	3	4	5
ENERGY	1	2	3	4	5
ACTIVITY	1	2	3	4	5
SLEEP	1	2	3	4	5

ANALYSIS OF SYMPTOM

DESCRIPTION	PAIN AREA

PAIN LEVEL

1	2	3	4	5	6	7	8	9	10

EXERCISE PLAN

	DESCRIPTION	DURATION / FREQUENCY
1		
2		
3		
4		
5		
6		
7		
8		
9		

📅 DATE		CLIENT CONDITIONS

📅 DATE	
🕐 TIME	
👤 CLIENT	
📅 AGE	
⚥ GENDER	

CLIENT CONDITIONS						
♥ HEALTH	1	2	3	4	5
⚡ ENERGY	1	2	3	4	5
🏃 ACTIVITY	1	2	3	4	5
🌙 SLEEP	1	2	3	4	5

ANALYSIS OF SYMPTOM

DESCRIPTION	PAIN AREA

PAIN LEVEL

1	2	3	4	5	6	7	8	9	10

EXERCISE PLAN

	DESCRIPTION	DURATION / FREQUENCY
1		
2		
3		
4		
5		
6		
7		
8		
9		

📅 DATE		CLIENT CONDITIONS					
🕐 TIME		💓 HEALTH	1	2	3	4	5
👤 CLIENT		⚡ ENERGY	1	2	3	4	5
📅 AGE		🏃 ACTIVITY	1	2	3	4	5
⚥ GENDER		🌙 SLEEP	1	2	3	4	5

ANALYSIS OF SYMPTOM

DESCRIPTION	PAIN AREA

PAIN LEVEL

1	2	3	4	5	6	7	8	9	10

EXERCISE PLAN

	DESCRIPTION	DURATION / FREQUENCY
1		
2		
3		
4		
5		
6		
7		
8		
9		

DATE		CLIENT CONDITIONS					
TIME		HEALTH	1	2	3	4	5
CLIENT		ENERGY	1	2	3	4	5
AGE		ACTIVITY	1	2	3	4	5
GENDER		SLEEP	1	2	3	4	5

ANALYSIS OF SYMPTOM

DESCRIPTION	PAIN AREA

PAIN LEVEL

1	2	3	4	5	6	7	8	9	10

EXERCISE PLAN

	DESCRIPTION	DURATION / FREQUENCY
1		
2		
3		
4		
5		
6		
7		
8		
9		

📅 DATE		**CLIENT CONDITIONS**					
🕐 TIME		〰️ HEALTH	1	2	3	4	5
👤 CLIENT		⚡ ENERGY	1	2	3	4	5
📆 AGE		🏃 ACTIVITY	1	2	3	4	5
⚥ GENDER		🌙 SLEEP	1	2	3	4	5

ANALYSIS OF SYMPTOM

DESCRIPTION	PAIN AREA

PAIN LEVEL

1	2	3	4	5	6	7	8	9	10

EXERCISE PLAN

	DESCRIPTION	DURATION / FREQUENCY
1		
2		
3		
4		
5		
6		
7		
8		
9		

DATE		CLIENT CONDITIONS					
TIME		HEALTH	1	2	3	4	5
CLIENT		ENERGY	1	2	3	4	5
AGE		ACTIVITY	1	2	3	4	5
GENDER		SLEEP	1	2	3	4	5

ANALYSIS OF SYMPTOM

DESCRIPTION	PAIN AREA

PAIN LEVEL

1	2	3	4	5	6	7	8	9	10

EXERCISE PLAN

	DESCRIPTION	DURATION / FREQUENCY
1		
2		
3		
4		
5		
6		
7		
8		
9		

📅 DATE		CLIENT CONDITIONS					
🕐 TIME		💓 HEALTH	1	2	3	4	5
👤 CLIENT		⚡ ENERGY	1	2	3	4	5
📅 AGE		🏃 ACTIVITY	1	2	3	4	5
⚥ GENDER		🌙 SLEEP	1	2	3	4	5

ANALYSIS OF SYMPTOM

DESCRIPTION	PAIN AREA

PAIN LEVEL

1	2	3	4	5	6	7	8	9	10

EXERCISE PLAN

	DESCRIPTION	DURATION / FREQUENCY
1		
2		
3		
4		
5		
6		
7		
8		
9		

📅 **DATE**		**CLIENT CONDITIONS**					
🕐 **TIME**		💓 HEALTH	1	2	3	4	5
🧍 **CLIENT**		⚡ ENERGY	1	2	3	4	5
📆 **AGE**		🏃 ACTIVITY	1	2	3	4	5
⚥ **GENDER**		🌙 SLEEP	1	2	3	4	5

ANALYSIS OF SYMPTOM

DESCRIPTION	PAIN AREA

PAIN LEVEL

1	2	3	4	5	6	7	8	9	10

EXERCISE PLAN

	DESCRIPTION	DURATION / FREQUENCY
1		
2		
3		
4		
5		
6		
7		
8		
9		

📅 DATE		CLIENT CONDITIONS

📅 DATE
🕐 TIME
🧍 CLIENT
📅 AGE
⚥ GENDER

CLIENT CONDITIONS					
❤️ HEALTH	1	2	3	4	5
⚡ ENERGY	1	2	3	4	5
🏃 ACTIVITY	1	2	3	4	5
🌙 SLEEP	1	2	3	4	5

ANALYSIS OF SYMPTOM

DESCRIPTION	PAIN AREA

PAIN LEVEL

1	2	3	4	5	6	7	8	9	10

EXERCISE PLAN

	DESCRIPTION	DURATION / FREQUENCY
1		
2		
3		
4		
5		
6		
7		
8		
9		

DATE		CLIENT CONDITIONS					
TIME		HEALTH	1	2	3	4	5
CLIENT		ENERGY	1	2	3	4	5
AGE		ACTIVITY	1	2	3	4	5
GENDER		SLEEP	1	2	3	4	5

ANALYSIS OF SYMPTOM

DESCRIPTION	PAIN AREA

PAIN LEVEL

1	2	3	4	5	6	7	8	9	10

EXERCISE PLAN

	DESCRIPTION	DURATION / FREQUENCY
1		
2		
3		
4		
5		
6		
7		
8		
9		

📅 DATE		CLIENT CONDITIONS	
🕐 TIME		💗 HEALTH	1 2 3 4 5
👤 CLIENT		⚡ ENERGY	1 2 3 4 5
📅 AGE		🏃 ACTIVITY	1 2 3 4 5
⚥ GENDER		🌙 SLEEP	1 2 3 4 5

ANALYSIS OF SYMPTOM

DESCRIPTION	PAIN AREA

PAIN LEVEL

1 2 3 4 5 6 7 8 9 10

EXERCISE PLAN

	DESCRIPTION	DURATION / FREQUENCY
1		
2		
3		
4		
5		
6		
7		
8		
9		

📅 DATE		CLIENT CONDITIONS					
🕐 TIME		💗 HEALTH	1	2	3	4	5
👤 CLIENT		⚡ ENERGY	1	2	3	4	5
📅 AGE		🏃 ACTIVITY	1	2	3	4	5
☿ GENDER		🌙 SLEEP	1	2	3	4	5

ANALYSIS OF SYMPTOM

DESCRIPTION	PAIN AREA

PAIN LEVEL

1	2	3	4	5	6	7	8	9	10

EXERCISE PLAN

	DESCRIPTION	DURATION / FREQUENCY
1		
2		
3		
4		
5		
6		
7		
8		
9		

	DATE		CLIENT CONDITIONS					
	TIME	HEALTH		1	2	3	4	5
	CLIENT	ENERGY		1	2	3	4	5
	AGE	ACTIVITY		1	2	3	4	5
	GENDER	SLEEP		1	2	3	4	5

ANALYSIS OF SYMPTOM

DESCRIPTION	PAIN AREA

PAIN LEVEL

1	2	3	4	5	6	7	8	9	10

EXERCISE PLAN

	DESCRIPTION	DURATION / FREQUENCY
1		
2		
3		
4		
5		
6		
7		
8		
9		

📅 **DATE**	
🕐 **TIME**	
👤 **CLIENT**	
📅 **AGE**	
⚥ **GENDER**	

CLIENT CONDITIONS

💓 HEALTH	1	2	3	4	5	
⚡ ENERGY	1	2	3	4	5	
🏃 ACTIVITY	1	2	3	4	5	
🌙 SLEEP	1	2	3	4	5	

ANALYSIS OF SYMPTOM

DESCRIPTION	PAIN AREA

PAIN LEVEL

1	2	3	4	5	6	7	8	9	10

EXERCISE PLAN

	DESCRIPTION	DURATION / FREQUENCY
1		
2		
3		
4		
5		
6		
7		
8		
9		

DATE		CLIENT CONDITIONS					
TIME		HEALTH	1	2	3	4	5
CLIENT		ENERGY	1	2	3	4	5
AGE		ACTIVITY	1	2	3	4	5
GENDER		SLEEP	1	2	3	4	5

ANALYSIS OF SYMPTOM

DESCRIPTION	PAIN AREA

PAIN LEVEL

1	2	3	4	5	6	7	8	9	10

EXERCISE PLAN

	DESCRIPTION	DURATION / FREQUENCY
1		
2		
3		
4		
5		
6		
7		
8		
9		

📅 **DATE**

🕐 **TIME**

👤 **CLIENT**

📇 **AGE**

⚧ **GENDER**

CLIENT CONDITIONS

〰️ HEALTH	1	2	3	4	5
〽️ ENERGY	1	2	3	4	5
🏃 ACTIVITY	1	2	3	4	5
🌙 SLEEP	1	2	3	4	5

ANALYSIS OF SYMPTOM

DESCRIPTION	PAIN AREA

PAIN LEVEL

| 1 | 2 | 3 | 4 | 5 | 6 | 7 | 8 | 9 | 10 |

EXERCISE PLAN

	DESCRIPTION	DURATION / FREQUENCY
1		
2		
3		
4		
5		
6		
7		
8		
9		

📅 DATE		CLIENT CONDITIONS					
🕐 TIME		〰️ HEALTH	1	2	3	4	5
👤 CLIENT		⚡ ENERGY	1	2	3	4	5
📅 AGE		🏃 ACTIVITY	1	2	3	4	5
⚥ GENDER		🌙 SLEEP	1	2	3	4	5

ANALYSIS OF SYMPTOM

DESCRIPTION	PAIN AREA

PAIN LEVEL

1	2	3	4	5	6	7	8	9	10

EXERCISE PLAN

	DESCRIPTION	DURATION / FREQUENCY
1		
2		
3		
4		
5		
6		
7		
8		
9		

📅 DATE		CLIENT CONDITIONS

🕐 TIME		❤️‍🩹 HEALTH	1	2	3	4	5

🧍 CLIENT		⚡ ENERGY	1	2	3	4	5

📅 AGE		🏃 ACTIVITY	1	2	3	4	5

⚥ GENDER		🌙 SLEEP	1	2	3	4	5

ANALYSIS OF SYMPTOM

DESCRIPTION	PAIN AREA

PAIN LEVEL

1	2	3	4	5	6	7	8	9	10

EXERCISE PLAN

	DESCRIPTION	DURATION / FREQUENCY
1		
2		
3		
4		
5		
6		
7		
8		
9		

📅 DATE		CLIENT CONDITIONS					
🕐 TIME		💗 HEALTH	1	2	3	4	5
👤 CLIENT		⚡ ENERGY	1	2	3	4	5
📅 AGE		🏃 ACTIVITY	1	2	3	4	5
⚤ GENDER		🌙 SLEEP	1	2	3	4	5

ANALYSIS OF SYMPTOM

DESCRIPTION	PAIN AREA

PAIN LEVEL

1	2	3	4	5	6	7	8	9	10

EXERCISE PLAN

	DESCRIPTION	DURATION / FREQUENCY
1		
2		
3		
4		
5		
6		
7		
8		
9		

📅 DATE		CLIENT CONDITIONS					
🕐 TIME		〰️ HEALTH	1	2	3	4	5
👤 CLIENT		⚡ ENERGY	1	2	3	4	5
📅 AGE		🏃 ACTIVITY	1	2	3	4	5
⚥ GENDER		🌙 SLEEP	1	2	3	4	5

ANALYSIS OF SYMPTOM

DESCRIPTION	PAIN AREA

PAIN LEVEL

1	2	3	4	5	6	7	8	9	10

EXERCISE PLAN

	DESCRIPTION	DURATION / FREQUENCY
1		
2		
3		
4		
5		
6		
7		
8		
9		

📅 DATE		CLIENT CONDITIONS	
🕐 TIME		❤️ HEALTH	⟨ 1 | 2 | 3 | 4 | 5 ⟩
👤 CLIENT		⚡ ENERGY	⟨ 1 | 2 | 3 | 4 | 5 ⟩
📅 AGE		🏃 ACTIVITY	⟨ 1 | 2 | 3 | 4 | 5 ⟩
⚥ GENDER		🌙 SLEEP	⟨ 1 | 2 | 3 | 4 | 5 ⟩

ANALYSIS OF SYMPTOM

DESCRIPTION	PAIN AREA

PAIN LEVEL

⟨ 1 \| 2 \| 3 \| 4 \| 5 \| 6 \| 7 \| 8 \| 9 \| 10 ⟩

EXERCISE PLAN

	DESCRIPTION	DURATION / FREQUENCY
1		
2		
3		
4		
5		
6		
7		
8		
9		

📅 **DATE**		
🕐 **TIME**		
👤 **CLIENT**		
📅 **AGE**		
⚢ **GENDER**		

CLIENT CONDITIONS

💓 HEALTH	1	2	3	4	5
⚡ ENERGY	1	2	3	4	5
🏃 ACTIVITY	1	2	3	4	5
🌙 SLEEP	1	2	3	4	5

ANALYSIS OF SYMPTOM

DESCRIPTION	PAIN AREA

PAIN LEVEL

1	2	3	4	5	6	7	8	9	10

EXERCISE PLAN

	DESCRIPTION	DURATION / FREQUENCY
1		
2		
3		
4		
5		
6		
7		
8		
9		

📅 DATE	
🕐 TIME	
👤 CLIENT	
📅 AGE	
⚧ GENDER	

CLIENT CONDITIONS

💓 HEALTH	1 2 3 4 5
⚡ ENERGY	1 2 3 4 5
🏃 ACTIVITY	1 2 3 4 5
🌙 SLEEP	1 2 3 4 5

ANALYSIS OF SYMPTOM

DESCRIPTION	PAIN AREA

PAIN LEVEL

1 2 3 4 5 6 7 8 9 10

EXERCISE PLAN

	DESCRIPTION	DURATION / FREQUENCY
1		
2		
3		
4		
5		
6		
7		
8		
9		

📅 DATE		CLIENT CONDITIONS					
🕐 TIME		❤️ HEALTH	1	2	3	4	5
👤 CLIENT		⚡ ENERGY	1	2	3	4	5
📅 AGE		🏃 ACTIVITY	1	2	3	4	5
⚧ GENDER		🌙 SLEEP	1	2	3	4	5

ANALYSIS OF SYMPTOM

DESCRIPTION	PAIN AREA

PAIN LEVEL

1	2	3	4	5	6	7	8	9	10

EXERCISE PLAN

	DESCRIPTION	DURATION / FREQUENCY
1		
2		
3		
4		
5		
6		
7		
8		
9		

📅 DATE	
🕐 TIME	
🧍 CLIENT	
📅 AGE	
⚥ GENDER	

CLIENT CONDITIONS

💗 HEALTH	1	2	3	4	5
⚡ ENERGY	1	2	3	4	5
🏃 ACTIVITY	1	2	3	4	5
🌙 SLEEP	1	2	3	4	5

ANALYSIS OF SYMPTOM

DESCRIPTION	PAIN AREA

PAIN LEVEL

1	2	3	4	5	6	7	8	9	10

EXERCISE PLAN

	DESCRIPTION	DURATION / FREQUENCY
1		
2		
3		
4		
5		
6		
7		
8		
9		

📅 DATE		CLIENT CONDITIONS					
🕐 TIME		❤️ HEALTH	1	2	3	4	5
👤 CLIENT		⚡ ENERGY	1	2	3	4	5
📅 AGE		🏃 ACTIVITY	1	2	3	4	5
⚥ GENDER		🌙 SLEEP	1	2	3	4	5

ANALYSIS OF SYMPTOM

DESCRIPTION	PAIN AREA

PAIN LEVEL

1	2	3	4	5	6	7	8	9	10

EXERCISE PLAN

	DESCRIPTION	DURATION / FREQUENCY
1		
2		
3		
4		
5		
6		
7		
8		
9		

📅 DATE		CLIENT CONDITIONS	
🕐 TIME		❤️ HEALTH	1 2 3 4 5
👤 CLIENT		⚡ ENERGY	1 2 3 4 5
📅 AGE		🏃 ACTIVITY	1 2 3 4 5
⚥ GENDER		🌙 SLEEP	1 2 3 4 5

ANALYSIS OF SYMPTOM

DESCRIPTION	PAIN AREA

PAIN LEVEL

1	2	3	4	5	6	7	8	9	10

EXERCISE PLAN

	DESCRIPTION	DURATION / FREQUENCY
1		
2		
3		
4		
5		
6		
7		
8		
9		

📅 DATE		CLIENT CONDITIONS					
🕐 TIME		💓 HEALTH	1	2	3	4	5
👤 CLIENT		⚡ ENERGY	1	2	3	4	5
📅 AGE		🏃 ACTIVITY	1	2	3	4	5
⚥ GENDER		🌙 SLEEP	1	2	3	4	5

ANALYSIS OF SYMPTOM

DESCRIPTION	PAIN AREA

PAIN LEVEL

1	2	3	4	5	6	7	8	9	10

EXERCISE PLAN

	DESCRIPTION	DURATION / FREQUENCY
1		
2		
3		
4		
5		
6		
7		
8		
9		

📅 DATE		CLIENT CONDITIONS	

📅 DATE
🕐 TIME
👤 CLIENT
📅 AGE
⚥ GENDER

CLIENT CONDITIONS

〽️ HEALTH		1 2 3 4 5
⚡ ENERGY		1 2 3 4 5
🏃 ACTIVITY		1 2 3 4 5
🌙 SLEEP		1 2 3 4 5

ANALYSIS OF SYMPTOM

DESCRIPTION	PAIN AREA

PAIN LEVEL

1	2	3	4	5	6	7	8	9	10

EXERCISE PLAN

	DESCRIPTION	DURATION / FREQUENCY
1		
2		
3		
4		
5		
6		
7		
8		
9		

		CLIENT CONDITIONS					
📅 DATE							
🕐 TIME	❤️ HEALTH	1	2	3	4	5	
👤 CLIENT	⚡ ENERGY	1	2	3	4	5	
📅 AGE	🏃 ACTIVITY	1	2	3	4	5	
⚥ GENDER	🌙 SLEEP	1	2	3	4	5	

ANALYSIS OF SYMPTOM

DESCRIPTION	PAIN AREA

PAIN LEVEL

1	2	3	4	5	6	7	8	9	10

EXERCISE PLAN

	DESCRIPTION	DURATION / FREQUENCY
1		
2		
3		
4		
5		
6		
7		
8		
9		

📅 DATE		CLIENT CONDITIONS					
🕐 TIME		〰️ HEALTH	1	2	3	4	5
👤 CLIENT		⚡ ENERGY	1	2	3	4	5
📅 AGE		🏃 ACTIVITY	1	2	3	4	5
⚥ GENDER		🌙 SLEEP	1	2	3	4	5

ANALYSIS OF SYMPTOM

DESCRIPTION	PAIN AREA

PAIN LEVEL

1	2	3	4	5	6	7	8	9	10

EXERCISE PLAN

	DESCRIPTION	DURATION / FREQUENCY
1		
2		
3		
4		
5		
6		
7		
8		
9		

📅 DATE		CLIENT CONDITIONS	
🕐 TIME		💓 HEALTH	1 2 3 4 5
👤 CLIENT		⚡ ENERGY	1 2 3 4 5
📅 AGE		🏃 ACTIVITY	1 2 3 4 5
⚥ GENDER		🌙 SLEEP	1 2 3 4 5

ANALYSIS OF SYMPTOM

DESCRIPTION	PAIN AREA

PAIN LEVEL

1 2 3 4 5 6 7 8 9 10

EXERCISE PLAN

	DESCRIPTION	DURATION / FREQUENCY
1		
2		
3		
4		
5		
6		
7		
8		
9		

📅 DATE		**CLIENT CONDITIONS**					
🕐 TIME		〰️ HEALTH	1	2	3	4	5
👤 CLIENT		⚡ ENERGY	1	2	3	4	5
📅 AGE		🏃 ACTIVITY	1	2	3	4	5
⚥ GENDER		🌙 SLEEP	1	2	3	4	5

ANALYSIS OF SYMPTOM

DESCRIPTION	PAIN AREA

PAIN LEVEL

1	2	3	4	5	6	7	8	9	10

EXERCISE PLAN

	DESCRIPTION	DURATION / FREQUENCY
1		
2		
3		
4		
5		
6		
7		
8		
9		

📅 DATE		CLIENT CONDITIONS	

📅 DATE	
🕐 TIME	
👤 CLIENT	
📅 AGE	
⚥ GENDER	

CLIENT CONDITIONS

❤️ HEALTH	1	2	3	4	5
⚡ ENERGY	1	2	3	4	5
🏃 ACTIVITY	1	2	3	4	5
🌙 SLEEP	1	2	3	4	5

ANALYSIS OF SYMPTOM

DESCRIPTION	PAIN AREA

PAIN LEVEL

1	2	3	4	5	6	7	8	9	10

EXERCISE PLAN

	DESCRIPTION	DURATION / FREQUENCY
1		
2		
3		
4		
5		
6		
7		
8		
9		

📅 DATE	
🕐 TIME	
👤 CLIENT	
📅 AGE	
⚥ GENDER	

CLIENT CONDITIONS

〰️ HEALTH	1	2	3	4	5
⚡ ENERGY	1	2	3	4	5
🏃 ACTIVITY	1	2	3	4	5
🌙 SLEEP	1	2	3	4	5

ANALYSIS OF SYMPTOM

DESCRIPTION	PAIN AREA

PAIN LEVEL

1	2	3	4	5	6	7	8	9	10

EXERCISE PLAN

	DESCRIPTION	DURATION / FREQUENCY
1		
2		
3		
4		
5		
6		
7		
8		
9		

📅 DATE	
🕐 TIME	
👤 CLIENT	
📅 AGE	
⚥ GENDER	

CLIENT CONDITIONS

〰️ HEALTH	1	2	3	4	5
⚡ ENERGY	1	2	3	4	5
🏃 ACTIVITY	1	2	3	4	5
🌙 SLEEP	1	2	3	4	5

ANALYSIS OF SYMPTOM

DESCRIPTION	PAIN AREA

PAIN LEVEL

1	2	3	4	5	6	7	8	9	10

EXERCISE PLAN

	DESCRIPTION	DURATION / FREQUENCY
1		
2		
3		
4		
5		
6		
7		
8		
9		

📅 DATE		**CLIENT CONDITIONS**					
🕐 TIME		❤️ HEALTH	1	2	3	4	5
👤 CLIENT		⚡ ENERGY	1	2	3	4	5
📅 AGE		🏃 ACTIVITY	1	2	3	4	5
⚥ GENDER		🌙 SLEEP	1	2	3	4	5

ANALYSIS OF SYMPTOM

DESCRIPTION	PAIN AREA

PAIN LEVEL

1	2	3	4	5	6	7	8	9	10

EXERCISE PLAN

	DESCRIPTION	DURATION / FREQUENCY
1		
2		
3		
4		
5		
6		
7		
8		
9		

	CLIENT CONDITIONS					
📅 DATE						
🕐 TIME	❤️ HEALTH	1	2	3	4	5
👤 CLIENT	⚡ ENERGY	1	2	3	4	5
📆 AGE	🏃 ACTIVITY	1	2	3	4	5
⚥ GENDER	🌙 SLEEP	1	2	3	4	5

ANALYSIS OF SYMPTOM

DESCRIPTION	PAIN AREA

PAIN LEVEL

1	2	3	4	5	6	7	8	9	10

EXERCISE PLAN

	DESCRIPTION	DURATION / FREQUENCY
1		
2		
3		
4		
5		
6		
7		
8		
9		

	DATE		CLIENT CONDITIONS					
	TIME		HEALTH	1	2	3	4	5
	CLIENT		ENERGY	1	2	3	4	5
	AGE		ACTIVITY	1	2	3	4	5
	GENDER		SLEEP	1	2	3	4	5

ANALYSIS OF SYMPTOM

DESCRIPTION	PAIN AREA

PAIN LEVEL

1	2	3	4	5	6	7	8	9	10

EXERCISE PLAN

	DESCRIPTION	DURATION / FREQUENCY
1		
2		
3		
4		
5		
6		
7		
8		
9		

📅 DATE		CLIENT CONDITIONS					
🕐 TIME		〰️ HEALTH	1	2	3	4	5
🧍 CLIENT		⚡ ENERGY	1	2	3	4	5
📆 AGE		🏃 ACTIVITY	1	2	3	4	5
⚥ GENDER		🌙 SLEEP	1	2	3	4	5

ANALYSIS OF SYMPTOM

DESCRIPTION	PAIN AREA

PAIN LEVEL

1	2	3	4	5	6	7	8	9	10

EXERCISE PLAN

	DESCRIPTION	DURATION / FREQUENCY
1		
2		
3		
4		
5		
6		
7		
8		
9		

📅 DATE		CLIENT CONDITIONS

📅 DATE	
🕐 TIME	
🧍 CLIENT	
📅 AGE	
⚧ GENDER	

CLIENT CONDITIONS

〜 HEALTH	1 2 3 4 5
⚡ ENERGY	1 2 3 4 5
🏃 ACTIVITY	1 2 3 4 5
🌙 SLEEP	1 2 3 4 5

ANALYSIS OF SYMPTOM

DESCRIPTION	PAIN AREA

PAIN LEVEL

1 2 3 4 5 6 7 8 9 10

EXERCISE PLAN

	DESCRIPTION	DURATION / FREQUENCY
1		
2		
3		
4		
5		
6		
7		
8		
9		

DATE		CLIENT CONDITIONS					
TIME		HEALTH	1	2	3	4	5
CLIENT		ENERGY	1	2	3	4	5
AGE		ACTIVITY	1	2	3	4	5
GENDER		SLEEP	1	2	3	4	5

ANALYSIS OF SYMPTOM

DESCRIPTION	PAIN AREA

PAIN LEVEL

1	2	3	4	5	6	7	8	9	10

EXERCISE PLAN

	DESCRIPTION	DURATION / FREQUENCY
1		
2		
3		
4		
5		
6		
7		
8		
9		

📅 DATE		CLIENT CONDITIONS					
🕐 TIME		〰️ HEALTH	1	2	3	4	5
👤 CLIENT		⚡ ENERGY	1	2	3	4	5
📅 AGE		🏃 ACTIVITY	1	2	3	4	5
⚥ GENDER		🌙 SLEEP	1	2	3	4	5

ANALYSIS OF SYMPTOM

DESCRIPTION	PAIN AREA

PAIN LEVEL

1	2	3	4	5	6	7	8	9	10

EXERCISE PLAN

	DESCRIPTION	DURATION / FREQUENCY
1		
2		
3		
4		
5		
6		
7		
8		
9		

📅 DATE		CLIENT CONDITIONS	
🕐 TIME		💓 HEALTH	1 2 3 4 5
🧑 CLIENT		⚡ ENERGY	1 2 3 4 5
📅 AGE		🏃 ACTIVITY	1 2 3 4 5
⚥ GENDER		🌙 SLEEP	1 2 3 4 5

ANALYSIS OF SYMPTOM

DESCRIPTION	PAIN AREA

PAIN LEVEL

| 1 | 2 | 3 | 4 | 5 | 6 | 7 | 8 | 9 | 10 |

EXERCISE PLAN

	DESCRIPTION	DURATION / FREQUENCY
1		
2		
3		
4		
5		
6		
7		
8		
9		

📅 DATE		**CLIENT CONDITIONS**	

📅 DATE	
🕐 TIME	
👤 CLIENT	
📅 AGE	
⚥ GENDER	

CLIENT CONDITIONS	
〰️ HEALTH	1 2 3 4 5
⚡ ENERGY	1 2 3 4 5
🏃 ACTIVITY	1 2 3 4 5
🌙 SLEEP	1 2 3 4 5

ANALYSIS OF SYMPTOM

DESCRIPTION	PAIN AREA

PAIN LEVEL

1 2 3 4 5 6 7 8 9 10

EXERCISE PLAN

	DESCRIPTION	DURATION / FREQUENCY
1		
2		
3		
4		
5		
6		
7		
8		
9		

DATE		CLIENT CONDITIONS					
TIME		HEALTH	1	2	3	4	5
CLIENT		ENERGY	1	2	3	4	5
AGE		ACTIVITY	1	2	3	4	5
GENDER		SLEEP	1	2	3	4	5

ANALYSIS OF SYMPTOM

DESCRIPTION

PAIN AREA

PAIN LEVEL

| 1 | 2 | 3 | 4 | 5 | 6 | 7 | 8 | 9 | 10 |

EXERCISE PLAN

	DESCRIPTION	DURATION / FREQUENCY
1		
2		
3		
4		
5		
6		
7		
8		
9		

📅 DATE		CLIENT CONDITIONS					
🕐 TIME		〰️ HEALTH	1	2	3	4	5
👤 CLIENT		⚡ ENERGY	1	2	3	4	5
📅 AGE		🏃 ACTIVITY	1	2	3	4	5
⚥ GENDER		🌙 SLEEP	1	2	3	4	5

ANALYSIS OF SYMPTOM

DESCRIPTION	PAIN AREA

PAIN LEVEL

1	2	3	4	5	6	7	8	9	10

EXERCISE PLAN

	DESCRIPTION	DURATION / FREQUENCY
1		
2		
3		
4		
5		
6		
7		
8		
9		

📅 DATE		CLIENT CONDITIONS	
🕐 TIME		〰 HEALTH	1 2 3 4 5
👤 CLIENT		⚡ ENERGY	1 2 3 4 5
📅 AGE		🏃 ACTIVITY	1 2 3 4 5
⚤ GENDER		🌙 SLEEP	1 2 3 4 5

ANALYSIS OF SYMPTOM

DESCRIPTION	PAIN AREA

PAIN LEVEL

1 2 3 4 5 6 7 8 9 10

EXERCISE PLAN

	DESCRIPTION	DURATION / FREQUENCY
1		
2		
3		
4		
5		
6		
7		
8		
9		

📅 DATE	
🕐 TIME	
👤 CLIENT	
📅 AGE	
⚥ GENDER	

CLIENT CONDITIONS

❤️ HEALTH	1	2	3	4	5
⚡ ENERGY	1	2	3	4	5
🏃 ACTIVITY	1	2	3	4	5
🌙 SLEEP	1	2	3	4	5

ANALYSIS OF SYMPTOM

DESCRIPTION	PAIN AREA

PAIN LEVEL

1	2	3	4	5	6	7	8	9	10

EXERCISE PLAN

	DESCRIPTION	DURATION / FREQUENCY
1		
2		
3		
4		
5		
6		
7		
8		
9		

DATE

TIME

CLIENT

AGE

GENDER

CLIENT CONDITIONS

HEALTH	1	2	3	4	5
ENERGY	1	2	3	4	5
ACTIVITY	1	2	3	4	5
SLEEP	1	2	3	4	5

ANALYSIS OF SYMPTOM

DESCRIPTION	PAIN AREA

PAIN LEVEL

| 1 | 2 | 3 | 4 | 5 | 6 | 7 | 8 | 9 | 10 |

EXERCISE PLAN

	DESCRIPTION	DURATION / FREQUENCY
1		
2		
3		
4		
5		
6		
7		
8		
9		

📅 DATE		CLIENT CONDITIONS	
🕐 TIME		❤️‍🩹 HEALTH	1 2 3 4 5
👤 CLIENT		⚡ ENERGY	1 2 3 4 5
📅 AGE		🏃 ACTIVITY	1 2 3 4 5
⚥ GENDER		🌙 SLEEP	1 2 3 4 5

ANALYSIS OF SYMPTOM

DESCRIPTION	PAIN AREA

PAIN LEVEL

1   2   3   4   5   6   7   8   9   10

EXERCISE PLAN

	DESCRIPTION	DURATION / FREQUENCY
1		
2		
3		
4		
5		
6		
7		
8		
9		

📅 DATE		CLIENT CONDITIONS

		CLIENT CONDITIONS					
📅 DATE		💓 HEALTH	1	2	3	4	5
🕐 TIME		⚡ ENERGY	1	2	3	4	5
👤 CLIENT		🏃 ACTIVITY	1	2	3	4	5
📅 AGE		🌙 SLEEP	1	2	3	4	5
⚥ GENDER							

ANALYSIS OF SYMPTOM

DESCRIPTION	PAIN AREA

PAIN LEVEL

1	2	3	4	5	6	7	8	9	10

EXERCISE PLAN

	DESCRIPTION	DURATION / FREQUENCY
1		
2		
3		
4		
5		
6		
7		
8		
9		

📅 DATE		**CLIENT CONDITIONS**					
🕐 TIME		〰️ HEALTH	1	2	3	4	5
👤 CLIENT		⚡ ENERGY	1	2	3	4	5
📅 AGE		🏃 ACTIVITY	1	2	3	4	5
⚥ GENDER		🌙 SLEEP	1	2	3	4	5

ANALYSIS OF SYMPTOM

DESCRIPTION	PAIN AREA

PAIN LEVEL

1	2	3	4	5	6	7	8	9	10

EXERCISE PLAN

	DESCRIPTION	DURATION / FREQUENCY
1		
2		
3		
4		
5		
6		
7		
8		
9		

📅 DATE		CLIENT CONDITIONS					
🕐 TIME		💓 HEALTH	1	2	3	4	5
🧍 CLIENT		⚡ ENERGY	1	2	3	4	5
📆 AGE		🏃 ACTIVITY	1	2	3	4	5
⚥ GENDER		🌙 SLEEP	1	2	3	4	5

ANALYSIS OF SYMPTOM

DESCRIPTION	PAIN AREA

PAIN LEVEL

1	2	3	4	5	6	7	8	9	10

EXERCISE PLAN

	DESCRIPTION	DURATION / FREQUENCY
1		
2		
3		
4		
5		
6		
7		
8		
9		

📅 DATE		CLIENT CONDITIONS					
🕐 TIME		〰 HEALTH	1	2	3	4	5
👤 CLIENT		⚡ ENERGY	1	2	3	4	5
📅 AGE		🏃 ACTIVITY	1	2	3	4	5
⚧ GENDER		🌙 SLEEP	1	2	3	4	5

ANALYSIS OF SYMPTOM

DESCRIPTION	PAIN AREA

PAIN LEVEL

1	2	3	4	5	6	7	8	9	10

EXERCISE PLAN

	DESCRIPTION	DURATION / FREQUENCY
1		
2		
3		
4		
5		
6		
7		
8		
9		

	DATE		CLIENT CONDITIONS					
	TIME		HEALTH	1	2	3	4	5
	CLIENT		ENERGY	1	2	3	4	5
	AGE		ACTIVITY	1	2	3	4	5
	GENDER		SLEEP	1	2	3	4	5

ANALYSIS OF SYMPTOM

DESCRIPTION	PAIN AREA

PAIN LEVEL

1	2	3	4	5	6	7	8	9	10

EXERCISE PLAN

	DESCRIPTION	DURATION / FREQUENCY
1		
2		
3		
4		
5		
6		
7		
8		
9		

Made in the USA
Las Vegas, NV
28 August 2022